the mystery of
masks

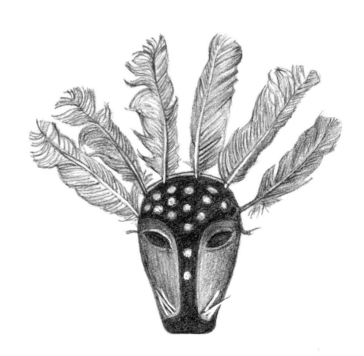

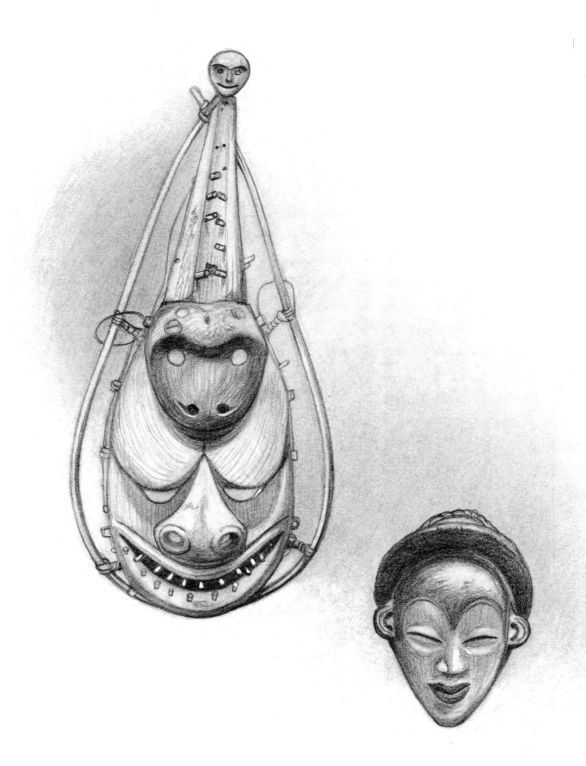

the mystery of
masks

by christine price

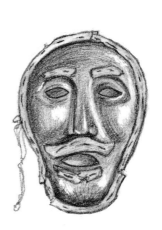

CHARLES SCRIBNER'S SONS

NEW YORK

Illustration on page 1:
ESKIMO MASK Alaska
Page 2:
Left: ESKIMO MASK Alaska
Right: AFRICAN MASK Gabon
Page 3: SIBERIAN MASK
Below: MEXICAN MASK
Opposite page: AFRICAN MASKS
Left: Cameroon *Right*: Zaire

This book is for Frank Waters

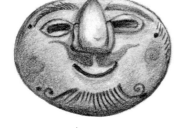

24611

Copyright © 1978 Christine Price
Library of Congress Cataloging in Publication Data
Price, Christine, 1928-
    The mystery of masks.
    SUMMARY: An illustrated overview of masks with
emphasis on their meaning and importance in each of the
cultures that produced them.
    1. Masks—Juvenile literature.   [1. Masks]
I. Title.
GN419.5.P74   392   77-27558
ISBN 0-684-15653-9
This book published simultaneously in the
United States of America and in Canada—
Copyright under the Berne Convention

1 3 5 7 9 11 13 15 17 19 MD/C 20 18 16 14 12 10 8 6 4 2
Printed in the United States of America

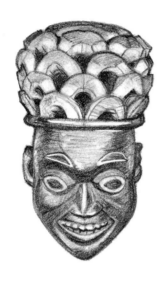

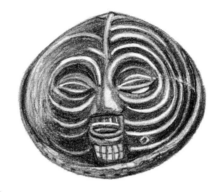

contents

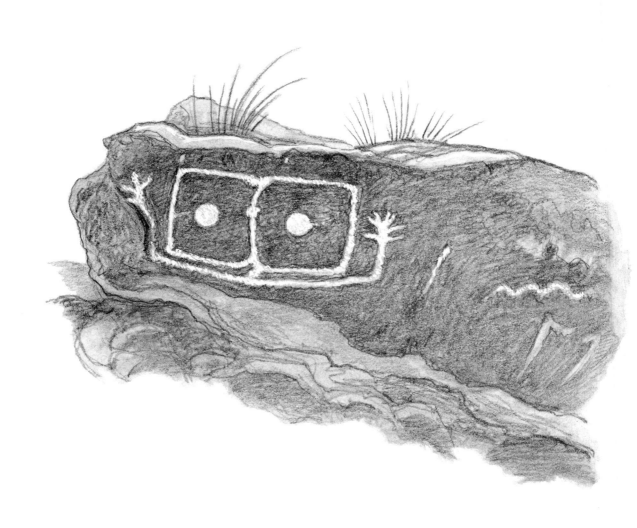

ROCK CARVINGS
New Mexico

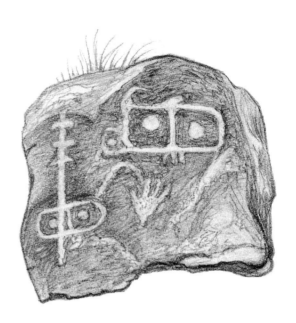

the power of masks

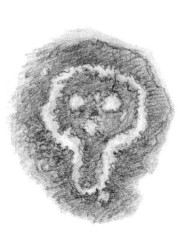

THEY stare at us from the rocks, the round-eyed masks, so old that no one knows who carved them there. Centuries of dust-laden winds have worn and weathered them; and the rocks have darkened under the hot sun and the swift slashing rains that send flash floods down the canyons and fill the dry pools with shining water. Are these the masks of gods, watching over the precious waterholes?

For the Pueblo Indians of this southwestern land, water has always been a holy thing. Rain comes as a gift from the gods, through prayer and ceremony and dance. Were the pools of water holy places to those people of long ago, the carvers of the rocks?

7

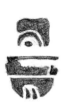

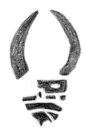

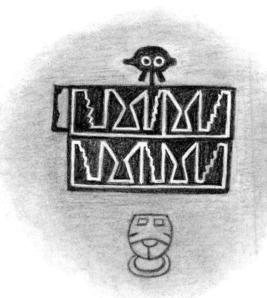

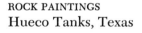

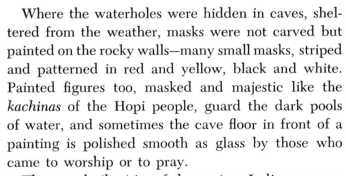

ROCK PAINTINGS
Hueco Tanks, Texas

Where the waterholes were hidden in caves, sheltered from the weather, masks were not carved but painted on the rocky walls—many small masks, striped and patterned in red and yellow, black and white. Painted figures too, masked and majestic like the *kachinas* of the Hopi people, guard the dark pools of water, and sometimes the cave floor in front of a painting is polished smooth as glass by those who came to worship or to pray.

The stonebuilt cities of the ancient Indians, ancestors of the Pueblo peoples of today, stand deserted and crumbling into ruin. A thousand years ago, when these were bustling places filled with life, the masked gods must have come at times of festival to spread

8

their blessing. Their images, mysterious and wonderful, were painted on the walls of *kivas*, the sacred rooms where men would gather for the rituals of their faith.

The *kiva* painters and the unknown artists of the rocks and caves knew the mystery of masks. They knew that the simplest mask could change the one who wore it into something new and strange, and that he who wore the mask of a god became the god himself.

KIVA PAINTING
Kuaua Pueblo, New Mexico

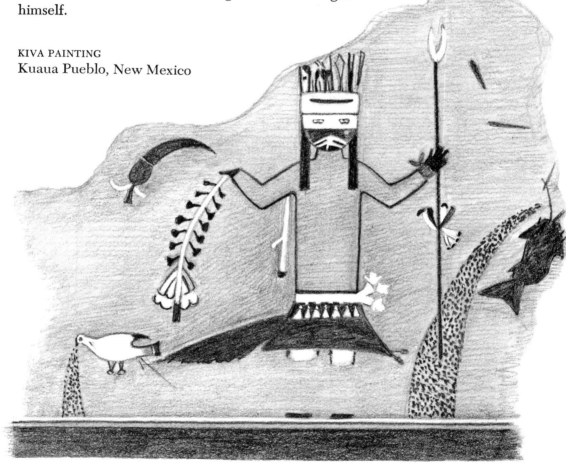

The people of ancient America were not alone in knowing the mysterious power of masks. Far away in northern Asia across the Bering Strait, masks were carved on the rocks of Siberia by prehistoric peoples. Masks appear among the Tassili rock paintings in the heart of the Sahara Desert. Masked figures dance on the walls of painted caves in India and in the rock paintings of southern Africa, the art of Bushman hunters. Even in the dark cave-sanctuaries of the Stone Age people of Europe there are pictures of dancing men in animal masks.

MASKS IN ANCIENT ROCK ART
Left: Siberia *Center*: India
Right: Tassili, North Africa
Opposite page:
Left: Bushman painting
Southern Africa
Right: Dancing shaman
Les Trois Frères cave, France

10

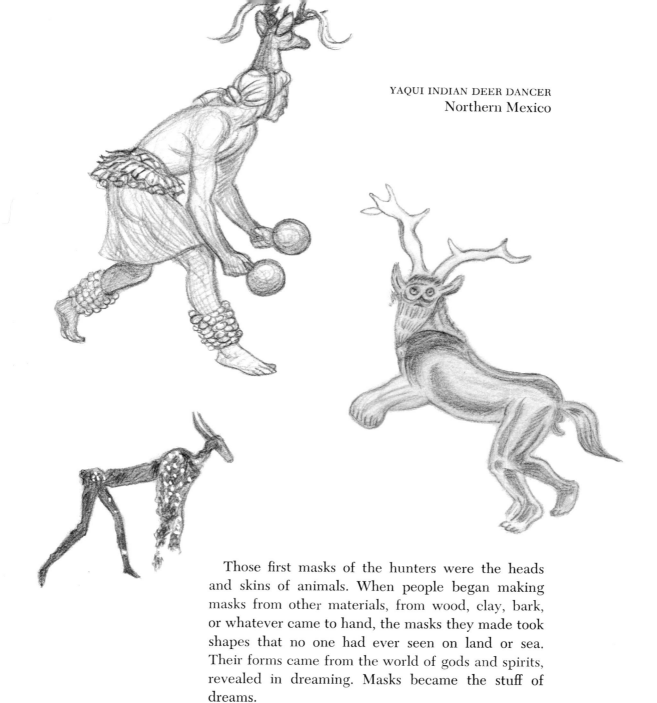

YAQUI INDIAN DEER DANCER
Northern Mexico

Those first masks of the hunters were the heads and skins of animals. When people began making masks from other materials, from wood, clay, bark, or whatever came to hand, the masks they made took shapes that no one had ever seen on land or sea. Their forms came from the world of gods and spirits, revealed in dreaming. Masks became the stuff of dreams.

11

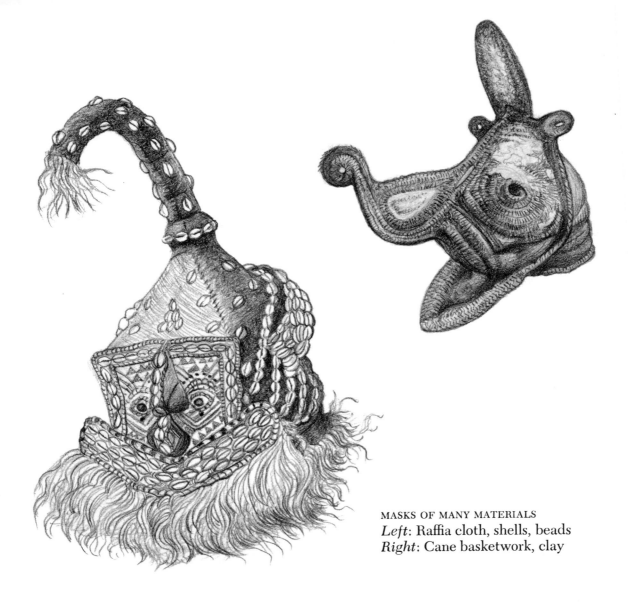

MASKS OF MANY MATERIALS
Left: Raffia cloth, shells, beads
Right: Cane basketwork, clay

Among hunting peoples, the dreamers were the shamans, men and women who possessed strange powers. In their dreams the shamans visited the spirit world, flew through the air like birds, and changed themselves from human beings to animals.

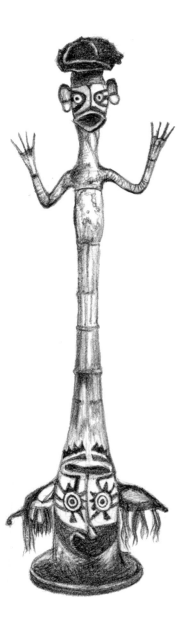

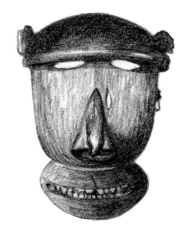

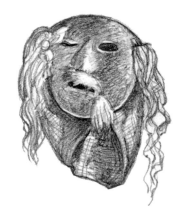

MASKS OF MANY MATERIALS
Left: Bark cloth, cane
Center: Wood
Right: Iron, cloth, bear fur

The shamans were the artists and the makers of masks. They led the people in ceremonies to bring success to the hunters. They could cure disease, curse evildoers, and give strength and wisdom to the children growing up.

When people began to farm the land and cultivate the plants they had gathered in the wild, new ceremonies of masks were linked with the seasons of the farmers' year. Masked gods presided over the times of planting and harvest. They blessed the fields with fruitfulness and the people with many children, and when a man or woman died, the masks of the ancestors would come to dance.

13

In towns and villages festivals were celebrated with sacred dramas, in which masked figures were the actors. The people watching, often in the courtyard of a temple, were drawn into a timeless world of dreams. They saw before their eyes the performance of mighty deeds by heroes of the past and even the exploits of the gods themselves. Demons fought with heroes in terrible battles of good and evil. Masked gods walked the earth, and to watch them was an act of prayer and praise.

As the centuries passed, some masks of the sacred dramas lost their holiness. In Europe, masks became mere entertainers. Seeing them make merry at Christmas or Mardi Gras, no one remembered what deep meaning they had had for people long ago.

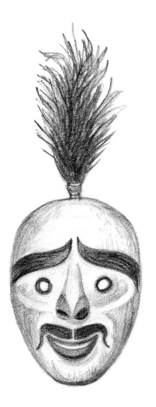
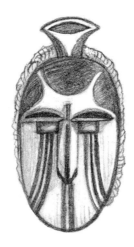
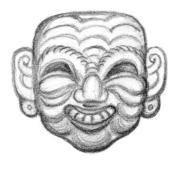

MASKS FOR DRAMA
Left: Canada, Kwakiutl people
Center: Africa, Afikpo people
Right: India, Monpa people

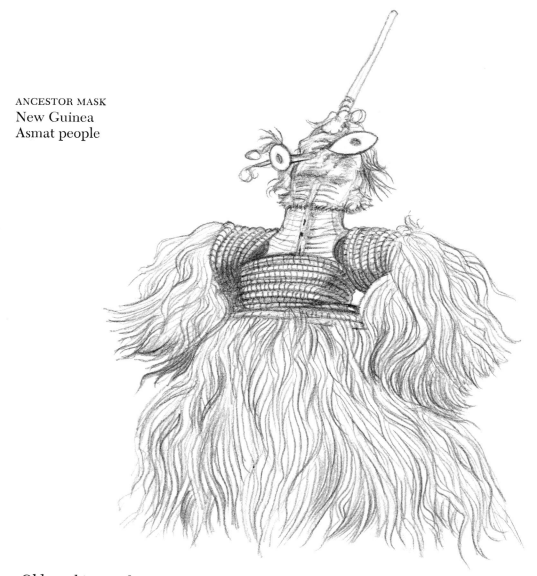

ANCESTOR MASK
New Guinea
Asmat people

Old masking traditions were often forgotten when peoples' lifeways changed. Village folk who moved to cities and struggled to earn a living could no longer spend months making masks and learning songs and dances for the great rituals of the year. When tribal peoples changed their faith and gave up their old gods, old ceremonies and the masks that went with them were quickly discarded.

Yet masks have never lost their mystery, that strange power that sets them apart from all other things that people have made. Even now, some masks are held sacred and kept hidden from prying eyes. We can still discover mask makers at work, filling the needs of their people, and the masks they make today reflect the dreams of ages past.

Deep in the countryside of West Bengal in India there is a village of mask makers, a cluster of earth-brown houses baking in the sun. If we go there in the spring, the mask makers will be busy preparing for the Spring Festival and the dramas of the Chhau Dance.

Every actor in the dance-dramas must have a mask. Many will play the parts of characters from the *Ramayana*, the epic story of the hero Rama and Sita, his beautiful wife. There are handsome white-painted faces for gods and heroes, masks of animals, and snarling faces of demons, colored brilliant green or red.

In villages for miles around, companies of dancers are rehearsing the old dramas, always performed when the land is waiting for the rains. The heat lies heavy on the fields and wooded hills. The soil has turned to dust, and dry leaves drop from the trees and crackle underfoot. But after the festival the rains will come . . .

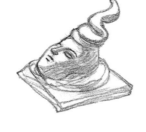

CHHAU MASKS AND
MASK MAKER
West Bengal, India

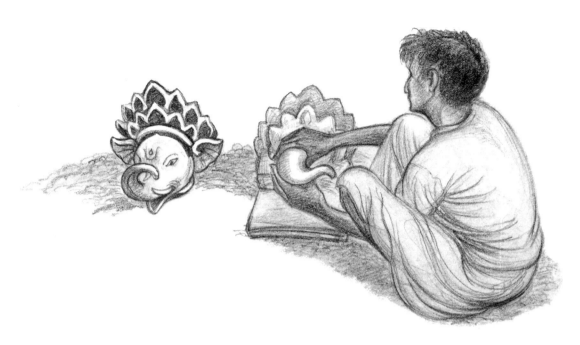

One of the mask makers, squatting in the dust outside his door, is shaping a mask of Ganesha, the cheerful, kindly god with the head of an elephant. Everyone loves Ganesha, and the Chhau Drama cannot begin without his blessing. He will be the first to appear on the night of the festival.

The craftsman works swiftly, modeling the mask of clay and strengthening it with thin layers of cloth and paper. After the head has been smoothed and dried, he will paint it gleaming white, the proper color for the god.

As we watch him at work on the elephant mask, we are carried back to the time of the Stone Age hunters, when the horned shaman danced the deer dance and animals were gods. The first masks were masks of animals, and their power has never been forgotten.

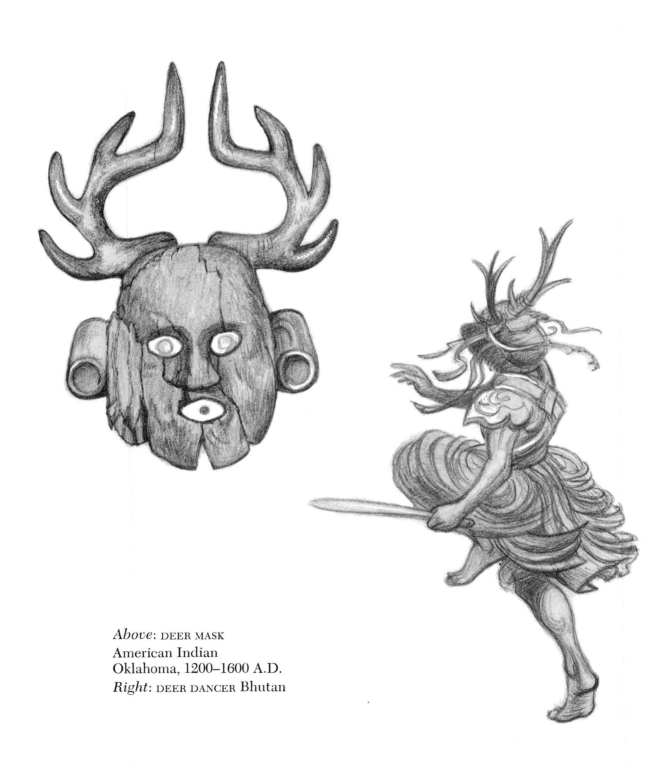

Above: DEER MASK
American Indian
Oklahoma, 1200–1600 A.D.
Right: DEER DANCER Bhutan

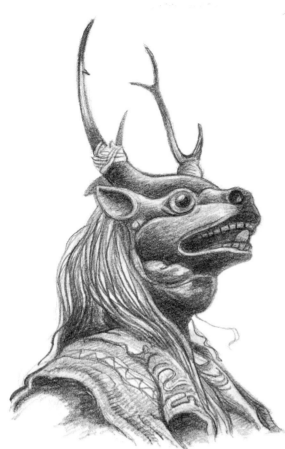

the animal world

HIGH in the Himalayas, in the small kingdom of Bhutan, the leaping deer dancer with his magic sword takes part in a Buddhist festival. His dance goes back to ancient times, long before the mountain peoples had heard the teachings of Buddha, but now he performs in the courtyard of a temple, to the music of clashing cymbals and thumping drums in the hands of Buddhist monks.

Eastward from Bhutan, in northern India, some of the mountain tribespeople are also followers of Buddha. Their old deer dances have developed into masked pantomimes that teach the Buddhist way. In the deer dance of the Sherdukpens, the hero Apapek and his two sons go hunting and catch a deer alive.

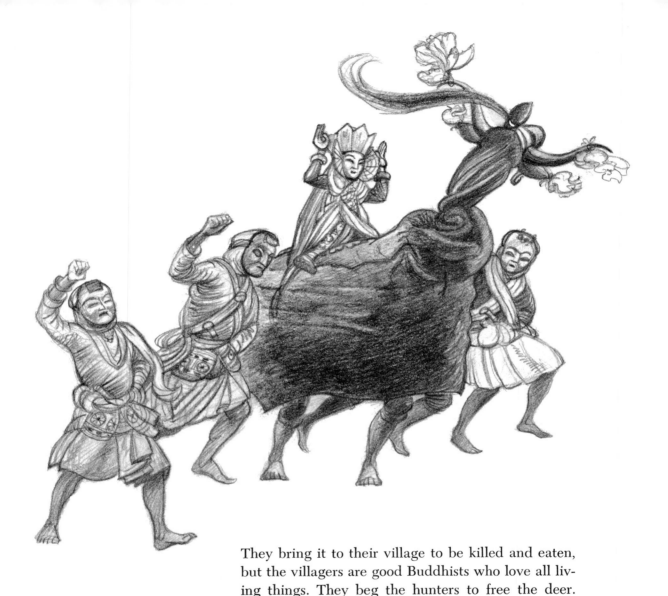

YAK DANCE
North India
Monpa people

They bring it to their village to be killed and eaten, but the villagers are good Buddhists who love all living things. They beg the hunters to free the deer. Their wish is granted, and the deer dances for joy.

Another favorite masked play of the Sherdukpens and their neighbors, the Monpas, tells the story of the yak, the hardy beast that provides the mountain folk with meat, milk, and butter. The first yak, so the story goes, was hatched from the egg of a mythical bird and discovered by one of the sons of Apapek.

In the final scene of the play, father and sons join the yak in a triumphant dance. With two men hidden inside its black cloth body, the yak prances on four lively legs, tossing its horned head and bearing on its back the carved figure of a beautiful goddess.

The yak, dancing with its captors, is a thoroughly domesticated animal. The African buffalo, on the other hand, is a wild creature of formidable strength. The horned buffalo masks made by peoples of West Africa were not meant for playacting. They were powerful in ceremonies to stamp out witchcraft and drive away evil spirits and, like most African masks, they could be worn only by members of secret societies. In the mask at the right, the buffalo head appears in its simplest form—little more than a pair of curved horns. These alone were a symbol of power.

BUFFALO MASKS
West Africa
Left: Ivory Coast
Baule people
Right: Nigeria
Mama people

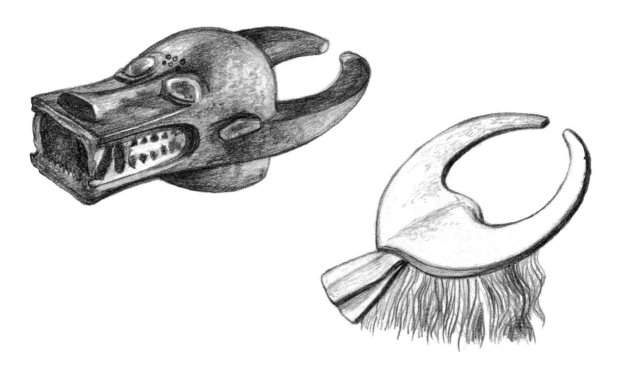

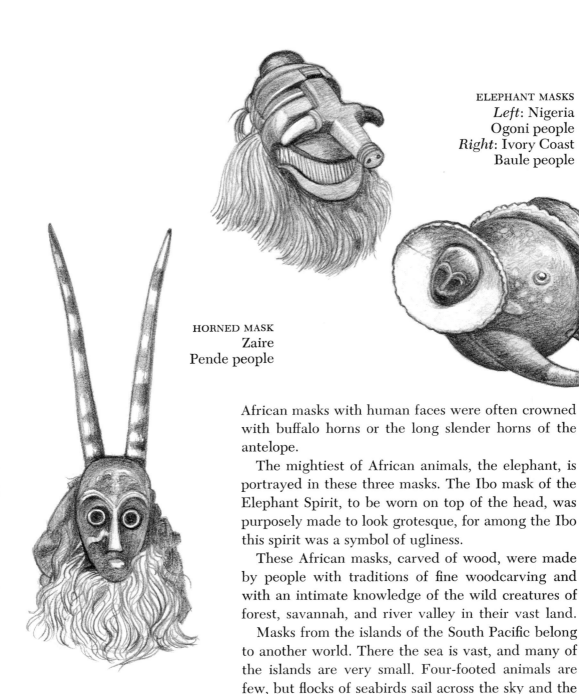

ELEPHANT MASKS
Left: Nigeria
Ogoni people
Right: Ivory Coast
Baule people

HORNED MASK
Zaire
Pende people

African masks with human faces were often crowned with buffalo horns or the long slender horns of the antelope.

The mightiest of African animals, the elephant, is portrayed in these three masks. The Ibo mask of the Elephant Spirit, to be worn on top of the head, was purposely made to look grotesque, for among the Ibo this spirit was a symbol of ugliness.

These African masks, carved of wood, were made by people with traditions of fine woodcarving and with an intimate knowledge of the wild creatures of forest, savannah, and river valley in their vast land.

Masks from the islands of the South Pacific belong to another world. There the sea is vast, and many of the islands are very small. Four-footed animals are few, but flocks of seabirds sail across the sky and the waters swarm with fish.

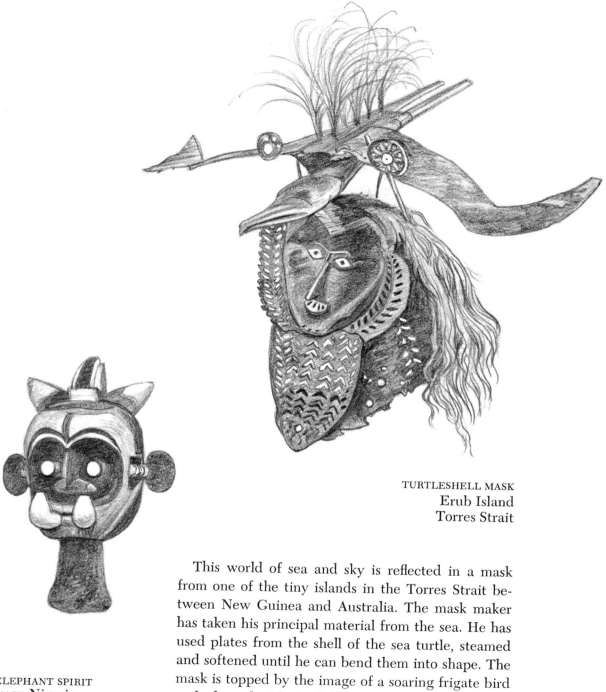

TURTLESHELL MASK
Erub Island
Torres Strait

ELEPHANT SPIRIT
MASK Nigeria
Ibo people

This world of sea and sky is reflected in a mask from one of the tiny islands in the Torres Strait between New Guinea and Australia. The mask maker has taken his principal material from the sea. He has used plates from the shell of the sea turtle, steamed and softened until he can bend them into shape. The mask is topped by the image of a soaring frigate bird and adorned with the delicate nodding plumes of the cassowary.

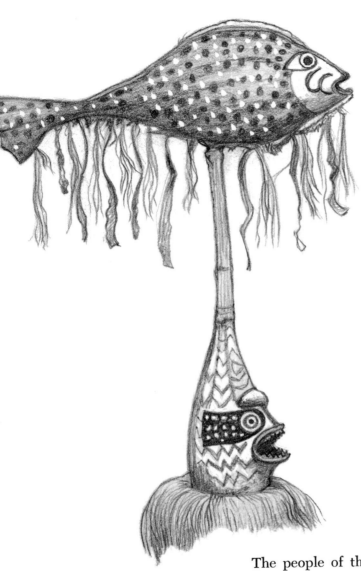

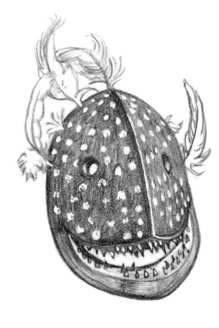

The people of the Papuan Gulf, on the northern side of the Torres Strait, made exciting masks from painted bark-cloth stretched on a framework of cane. This one was worn for clowning and making fun during a long and solemn religious festival. The spotted fish that crowns the mask represents a sacred animal, the mythical ancestor of a tribal clan.

A fat blackfish tufted with feathers and a splendid

FISH MASKS
Left: Papuan Gulf
Right: Alaska
Eskimo

24

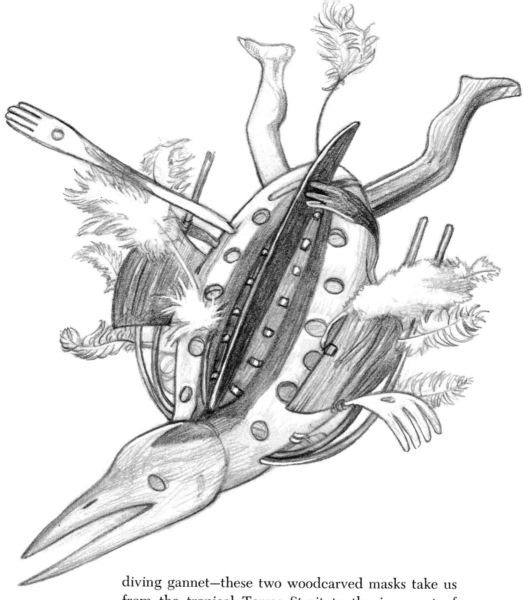

diving gannet—these two woodcarved masks take us from the tropical Torres Strait to the icy coast of Alaska. The Pacific islanders of the warm south could live by farming as well as fishing, but for the Alaskan Eskimos, sea people of the north, hunting and fishing were the only ways to survive. Their lives depended on the hunters' skill, but also on the hunting magic of the shamans and the power of masks.

GANNET MASK
Alaska, Eskimo

25

The Eskimo masks, carved of driftwood, were never copies of the familiar forms of beasts and birds. They were shaped by the shamans' dreams.

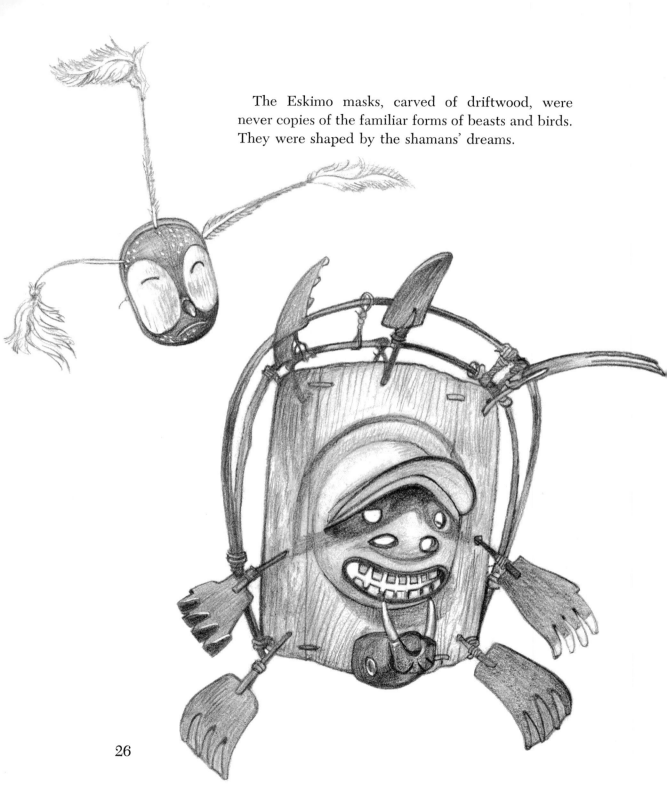

The carver of the gannet mask has shown the bird diving into the sea after a fish, as gannets do; but this bird has human feet and hands, and inside its hollow head is a tiny human face—the gannet's soul.

In the Eskimo's world, all living creatures had souls. The souls of animals were the spirit-helpers of the shamans, seen in dreams and made visible in the shamans' masks. The souls of animals killed for food were not forgotten by the Eskimo hunters. When they brought home a seal or a walrus, they would save its bladder, believed to be the dwelling of the soul. The bladders were displayed each year at the Bladder Festival in November, when the people honored the dead animals with dances in animal masks and prayed for good hunting in the year to come. Then the seal bladders were taken back to the sea so that the dead seals might come alive again.

The little owl mask with the three plumes was made for dancing at the Bladder Festival. The fierce owl mask below, deeply carved, was for dances of the Kwakiutl Indians of the northwest coast.

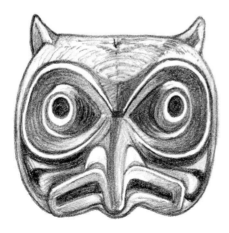

Opposite page:
Left: OWL MASK
Right: SHAMAN'S MASK
OF WALRUS SPIRIT
Both Alaskan Eskimo

OWL MASK
British Columbia, Kwakiutl people

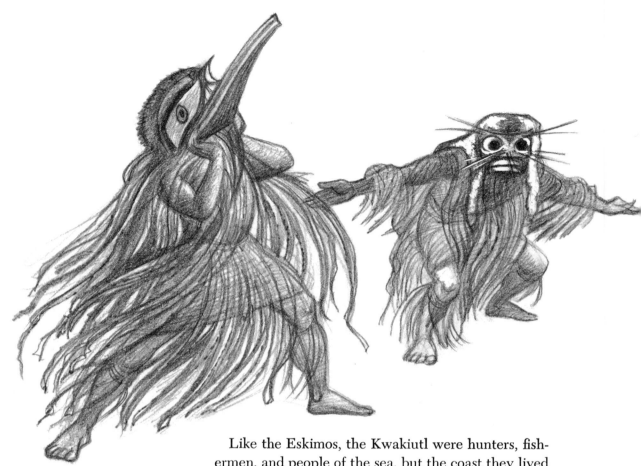

DANCERS IN
HAMATSA CEREMONY
Left: Raven
Right: Wasp
Opposite page:
Crooked-Beak-of-the-Sky

Like the Eskimos, the Kwakiutl were hunters, fishermen, and people of the sea, but the coast they lived on, around the northern end of Vancouver Island, was not the bare tundra country that the Eskimo knew. Dense evergreen forests came down to the shore. There was unlimited wood for the carver, and the Kwakiutl were brilliant artists in wood. Above all, they were makers of masks.

Scores of wooden masks were needed for the great dance-dramas staged in the houses of chiefs when winter storms lashed the coast and the people were glad to be indoors. Winter was the sacred time. Ancient tales were retold, and terrible and wonderful figures from the misty past came alive before the people's eyes in the dancing of the masks.

28

The huge masks of Raven and Crooked-Beak-of-the-Sky would dance at the initiation ceremonies for a new member of the Hamatsa, the secret society of the Cannibal Spirit. They were Cannibal Birds, servants of the spirit. In the shadowy hall of the chief's house, they would appear from behind a painted wooden screen and dance in the firelight, swinging their mighty beaks and opening and shutting them with a dreadful clacking sound. The young man to be initiated was in a state of frenzy after many days of fasting in the forest, the home of the Cannibal Spirit. The masks danced to calm him.

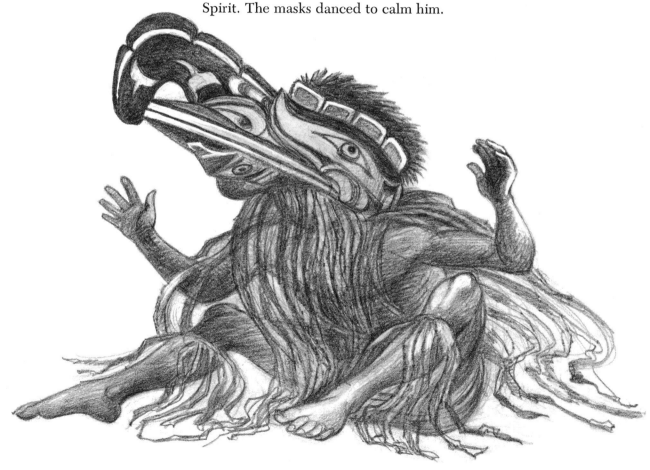

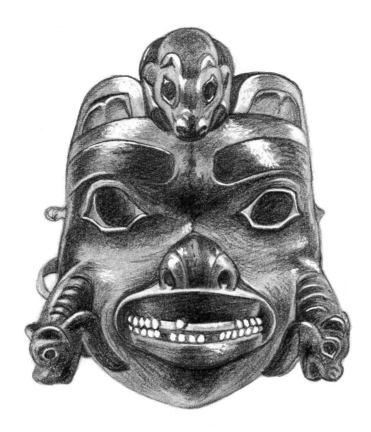

SHAMAN'S MASK
OF BEAR SPIRIT
Alaska, Tlingit people

Fresh masks appeared and whirled in the firelight
to the chant of sacred songs and the beat of the drum
until at last the new Hamatsa was ready to come
forth and dance before his people.

To those who watched the ceremonies, the masks
of birds, beasts, insects, and monsters were more
than actors in a play. They were a living part of the
everyday world. For the Kwakiutl, there was no
boundary between animals and people. The Indians
traced their families back to animal ancestors, to
Bear, Raven, Wolf, and Thunderbird. Humans and
animals could change their shapes, and many masks
were carved in forms half animal, half human.

The snarling mask above, a mixture of bear and
man, belonged to a shaman of the Tlingit people,

30

Indians of the coast of Alaska. Shamans were powerful among the Indians, not only in the northwest but throughout the Americas. This northern shaman had a bear for his helping spirit; in the tropical forests of Central and South America he might have changed himself into a jaguar.

The ancient peoples of Mexico worshipped the jaguar as a god, and in Mexico today, jaguar masks are still made for traditional animal dances. The dancer below, in his mask and spotted costume, is taking the lead in the "Dance of the Tiger." This is a comic pantomime about a band of frightened hunters out to kill a jaguar; but its roots are deep in the Indian past when the jaguar was the god of the earth and brought fertility to the farmers' fields of corn.

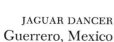

ANCIENT OLMEC
CARVING Mexico

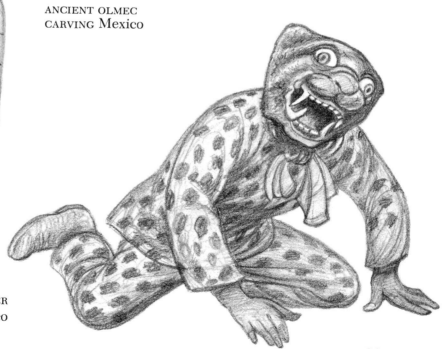

JAGUAR DANCER
Guerrero, Mexico

31

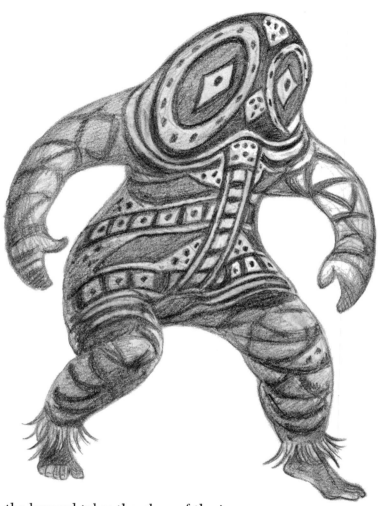

LEOPARD DANCER
Cameroon
Kaka people

In Africa, the leopard takes the place of the jaguar. Strong and beautiful, he is the symbol of kingship and of the power to do great things.

This leopard costume, covering the dancer from head to foot with a sinuous patterned skin, was worn by members of a Leopard Society in Cameroon, hunters who performed a leopard dance before and after the hunt.

The leopard is a matchless hunter. He appears, carved in wood, on the top of a mask from Nigeria, springing out with bared teeth to attack a snake.

This is one of many masks made for the Egungun Society of the Yoruba people. They represent the spirits of ancestors, the heroes of the past. Some of the masks are made of wood like this one, with human faces and often with the long pointed ears of an animal. Others, called "The Children of Egungun," are strange faceless beings, neither animal nor human. They are spirit-visions from another world, and to see them is to feel again the mysterious power of masks.

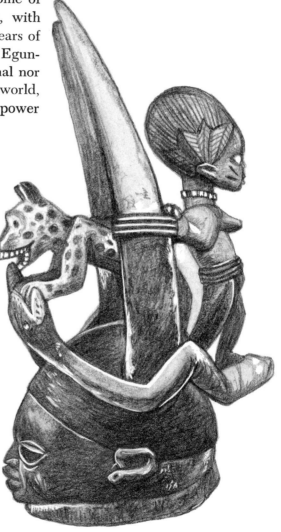

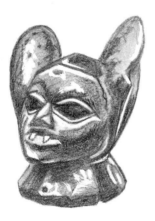

EGUNGUN MASKS
Nigeria, Yoruba people

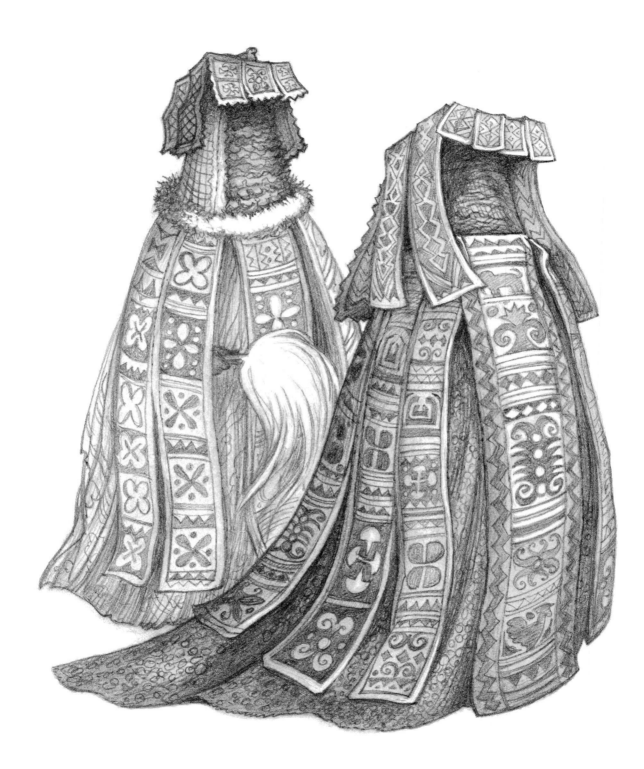

spirits and human beings

THE Egungun masks come silently gliding, robed in brilliant colors, fit for a king. The scene of their coming may be a West African city, loud with the roar of traffic, or a little mudwalled village in a grove of palms; but wherever the Egungun are seen, no one dares come near them. People draw back in awe to let them pass, for these are visitors from the spirit world, the spirits of long-dead kings.

Their royalty and their unearthliness are expressed in the glowing costumes. The many strips of material, covered with appliqué designs, swirl around them in a rainbow of color when the Egungun begin to dance.

Through the magic of masks, these and a host of other spirits can come to earth and visit the people. Wherever they appear, their forms are mysterious and wonderful.

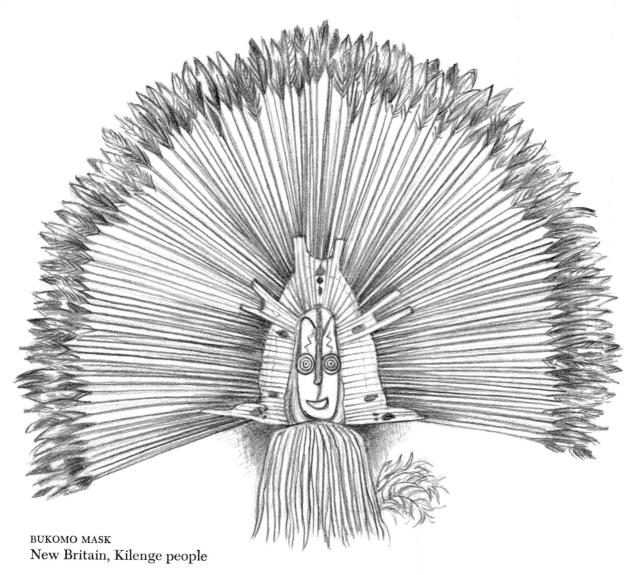

BUKOMO MASK
New Britain, Kilenge people

On the island of New Britain in the South Pacific the tall mask called Bukomo, with its swaying feathered crown, stalks through the villages of the Kilenge people. It comes to preside over the ear-piercing ceremony, an important event in the lives of young boys growing up. The owl-eyed mask, also from New Britain, represents a kindly spirit that protects little children, while the Bundu mask from West Africa—

one of the few masks worn by women—serves as a teacher of young girls preparing for womanhood. Bundu masks always show the face of a beautiful woman with a high forehead and elegant hairstyle, reminding the girls of what they will be when they grow up.

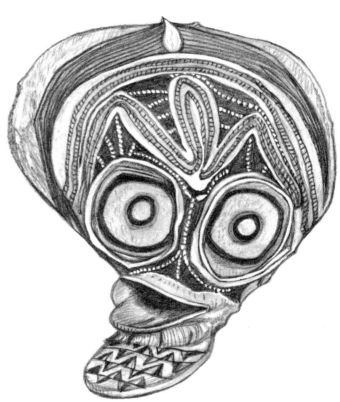

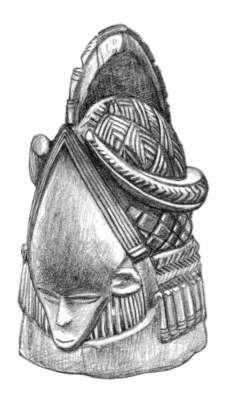

Left: BUNDU MASK
Sierra Leone
Mende people
Right: OWL MASK
New Britain
Baining people

37

Among many peoples throughout the world the time of growing up and leaving childhood behind is marked by elaborate ceremonies of initiation. This is a time of learning and testing, but also of danger, calling for the protection and guidance of gods and spirits. The African mask below, worn for dances after the initiation of boys of the Pende people, represents an important human being rather than a spirit, but it is believed to have power over the forces of the spirit world.

INITIATION MASK
Zaire, Pende people

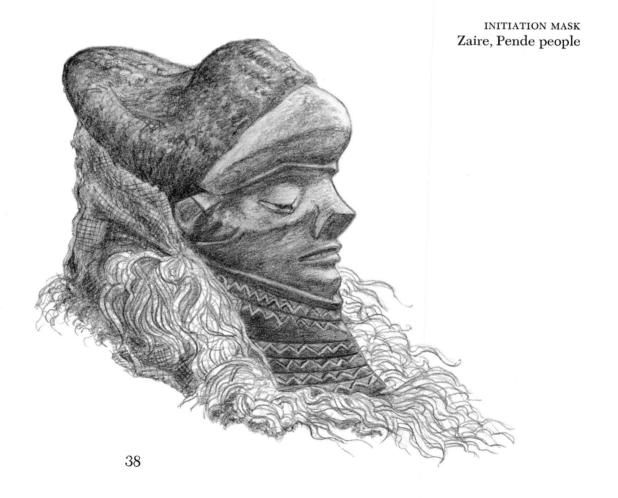

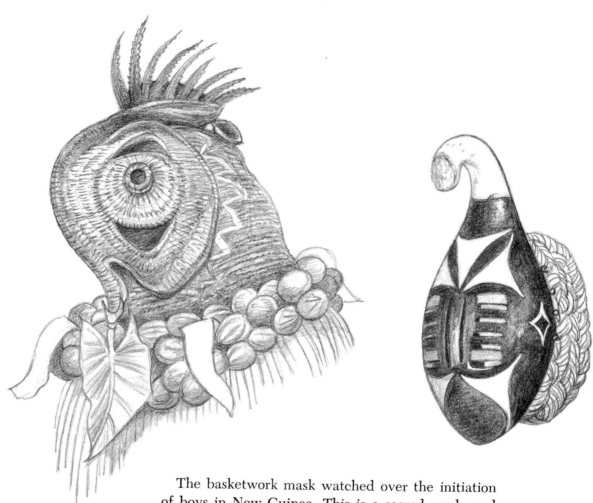

The basketwork mask watched over the initiation of boys in New Guinea. This is a sacred mask, and women and children are forbidden to look on its birdlike face.

The mask from the Afikpo people of Nigeria is also sacred and kept hidden when not in use. Masks like this one, made from hollow painted gourds, are worn by the eldest sons of important families when they are accepted as members of a men's secret society. The natural shape of the gourd gives its form to the mask, and there is no attempt to make it look like a human face. But in the dream world of masks, even human faces can take strange forms.

INITIATION MASKS
Left: Sepik River
Papua New Guinea
Right: Nigeria
Afikpo people

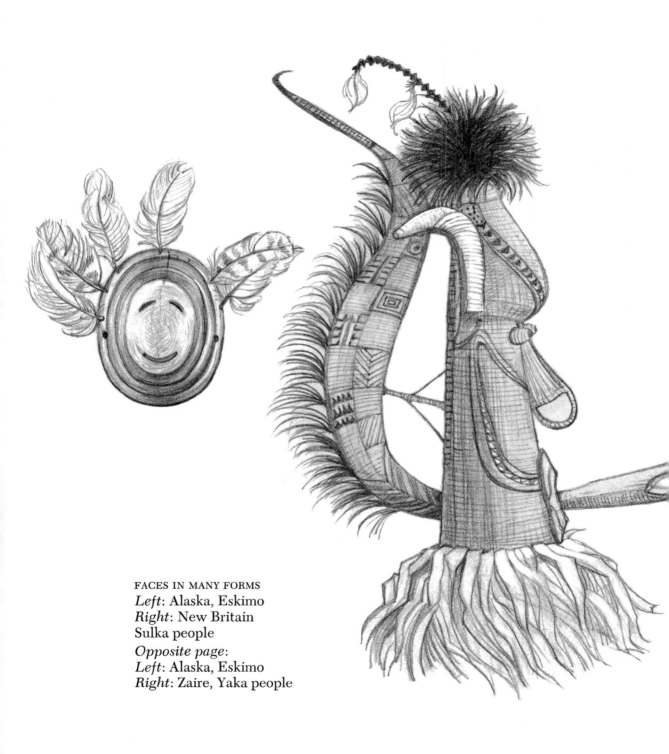

FACES IN MANY FORMS
Left: Alaska, Eskimo
Right: New Britain
Sulka people
Opposite page:
Left: Alaska, Eskimo
Right: Zaire, Yaka people

Faces may be squat and round, or tall and thin. The feathered Eskimo mask has eyes and mouth but no nose. The African mask below has a nose that juts out like the trunk of an elephant.

Not all these masks have deep meaning and a serious intent. The big-nosed one is for fun and celebration. It would be worn with pride by a boy of the Yaka people, after the ordeals of his initiation were over. He and other boys who had newly come to manhood would dance through the villages, showing off their masks to everyone.

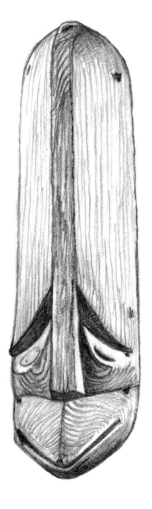

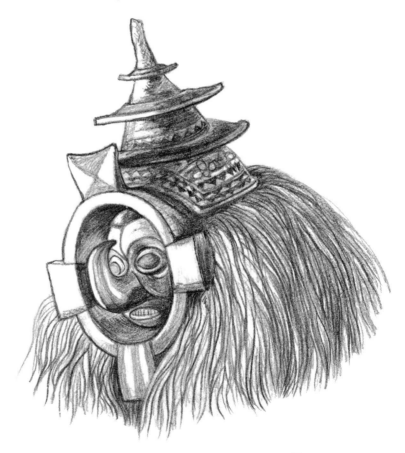

Big noses are also a feature of the Kwakiutl masks called Fool Dancers, whose task was to keep order among the people at the winter drama of the Cannibal Spirit.

Some masks make fun on solemn occasions. The Japanese one opposite was used in Kyogen, the short plays that provide comic relief in a program of Noh, the stately masked drama of Japan.

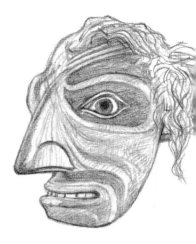

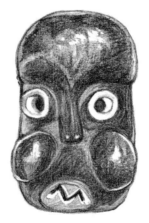

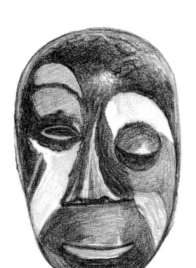

Left and center:
DRAMA MASKS
Nigeria, Afikpo people
Right:
MASK OF FOOL
DANCER
British Columbia
Kwakiutl people

42

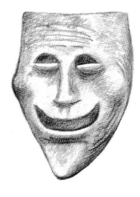

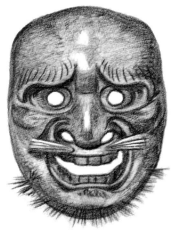

Left: CLOWN MASK
Guerrero, Mexico

Center: COMEDY MASK
Japan

Right: MASK FOR
DANCE-DRAMA Korea

   Masks can also criticize and poke fun at proud and pompous people, and those who pretend to be better than they are. The black masks opposite, called "ugly faces" by the Afikpo people who make them, represent greedy selfish old men in the Afikpo plays. The white hairy mask at the right appears in dance-dramas of Korea, playing the part of a rich landowner of noble birth and quite astonishing stupidity.

43

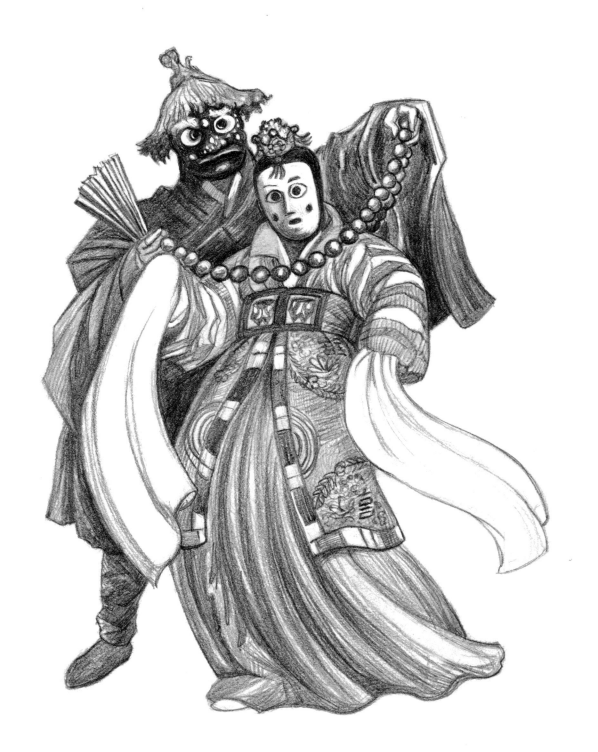

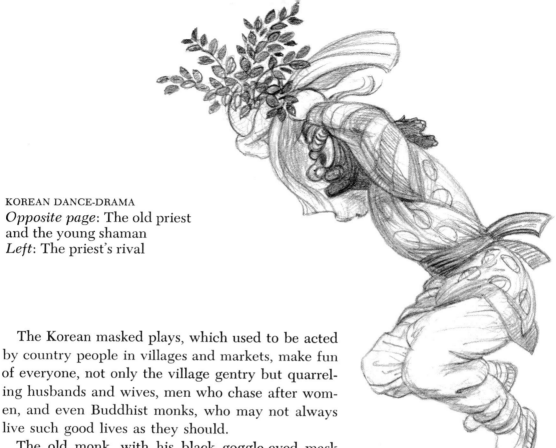

KOREAN DANCE-DRAMA
Opposite page: The old priest
and the young shaman
Left: The priest's rival

The Korean masked plays, which used to be acted by country people in villages and markets, make fun of everyone, not only the village gentry but quarreling husbands and wives, men who chase after women, and even Buddhist monks, who may not always live such good lives as they should.

The old monk, with his black goggle-eyed mask and comical straw hat, is a stock character. He falls in love with a beautiful young woman, and when she sternly rejects him, he tries to persuade her by putting his big wooden rosary around her neck.

The young woman is portrayed as a shaman, for shamans, usually women, were important in Korea in the past. The masked plays had their beginnings in the masked dances of shamans. The fierce black mask of the old monk and the red one of the young man, his rival in love, were originally powerful masks used by shamans for ceremonies of curing. To cure sickness meant driving out the demons that caused it, and to do this the shaman would dance in a demon mask.

45

The old belief in sickness-demons and in curing by the power of masks is still alive today.

In North America, the False Face masks of the Iroquois show the distorted face of the demon that first brought sickness to the Indians. Members of the False Face Society make their own masks for the winter ceremonies of curing illness and casting out evil. Each man carves the mask according to his own vision. The False Faces are sacred, and in the past they were carved only from living trees.

The grinning demon mask comes from the island of Sri Lanka, at the southern tip of India, where a whole crowd of demons are believed to be responsible for different diseases. The mask of the cross-eyed man was used in curing dances of the Monpa in

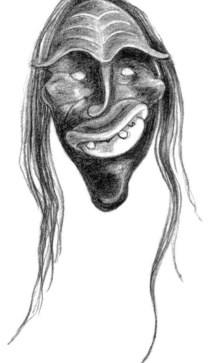

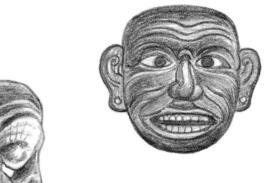

MASKS FOR CURING
Left: Iroquois False Face
Onondaga, New York
Center: Devil mask
Sri Lanka
Right: Cross-eyed mask
North India, Monpa people

46

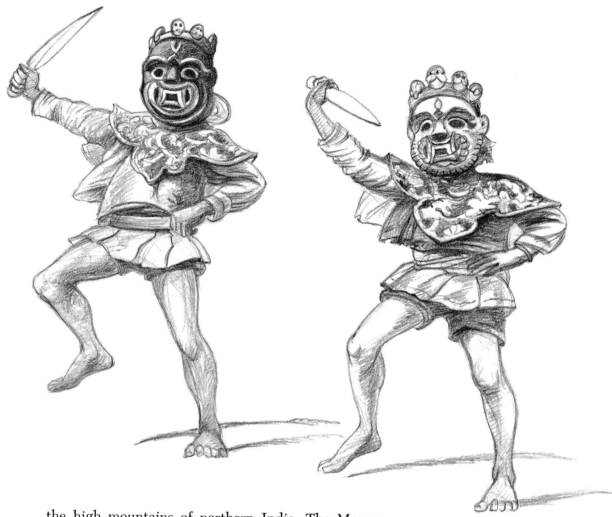

the high mountains of northern India. The Monpa and their neighbors are Buddhists, as we have seen. Demons, to them, are the enemies of Buddhism. Their masked pantomimes dramatize the mythical battles between the demons and the equally ferocious spirits that defend the people and their faith.

The belief in demons, the enemies of gods and men, has inspired some thrilling masked dramas that bring to life, for all to see, the never-ending war between good and evil.

DANCE OF
GOOD SPIRITS
North India

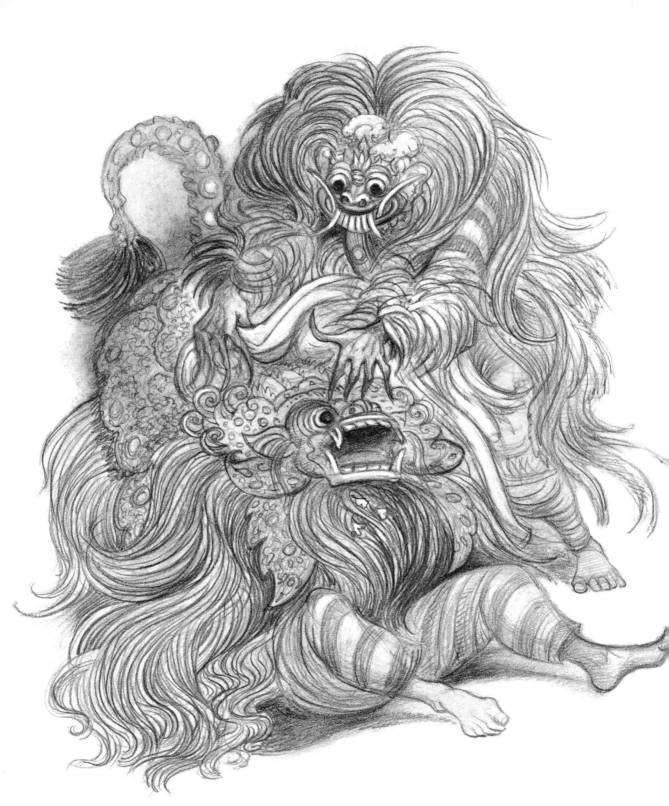

demons, gods, and heroes

A BATTLE rages in a temple courtyard under the night sky of Bali. Hideous Rangda the witch, the bringer of all evil, fights against the great beast Barong, the champion and defender of the people.

Now she bears down on him, pressing him to the ground. The light of the flaring torches gleams on her keen fangs and lolling tongue, glaring eyes and tangled mane of hair. The music of the *gamelan* quickens, with the rapid heartbeat of the drum and the sharp repeated patterns of cymbals and bell-like gongs.

A crowd of people crouches on the ground to watch the battle, seen so many times before yet always new. The man who wears the witch mask and

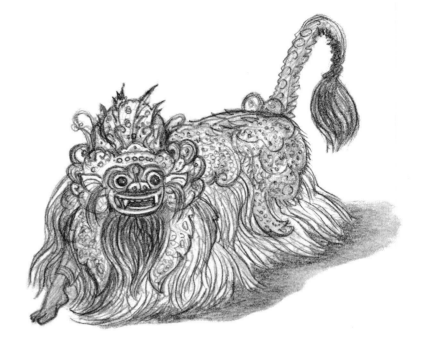

BARONG
Bali

the two men hidden in the huge glistening body of the Barong fight in trance, possessed by the strong spirits of the two eternal enemies. Even some of the watching people are seized by the spirits. Staggering in trance around the temple court, men stab themselves with knives and feel no pain.

From the richly carved gateways and walls of the temple the sculptured figures of the gods look on at the scene of battle, and in the torchlight their images seem to dance. These are gods of the Hindu faith that came to Bali from India many centuries ago— Vishnu and Shiva, the mother goddess Durga and cheerful Ganesha with the head of an elephant.

The same gods watch over the people in faraway villages in West Bengal, in the heart of India. There too the war between good and evil is fought out under the stars, but not by Rangda and Barong. The fighters are the demons, gods, and heroes of the Chhau Dance, and the time of their battle is the Spring Festival, when the land waits for the rains.

50

By nightfall on the first day of the festival companies of dancers from villages far and near have arrived at the festival grounds. They come on foot with drummers pounding on their drums, and the precious masks, newly made in the village of the mask makers, are carried shoulder-high on long wooden litters.

Hundreds of people surround the dancing place, crushed together up the slope of the hillside and perched in the trees above. Ropes have been stretched around a square space of bare earth and along the sides of the passageway leading down to it, where the dancers will enter. Lanterns, hanging on poles, shed a brilliant light on the dancing place.

The drummers are already assembled. Three men sit behind the big bowl-shaped *dhamsa* drums, and two parade about playing softly on the long *dhol* drums slung from their shoulders. A boy sings in a high thin voice an invocation to Ganesha, the god who will open the festival. Then suddenly the big drums begin to boom and the smaller ones to crackle and clatter. The *dhol* drummers prance in a circle, then run to the entrance of the passageway, shouting hoarsely into the darkness, as though they were calling spirits from the forest. Where is Ganesha? Was that a glimmer of brightness in the dark?

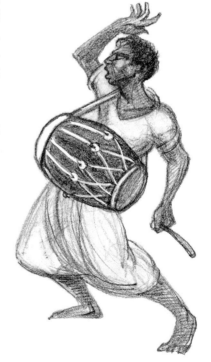

DHOL DRUMMER
AT THE CHHAU DANCE
West Bengal, India

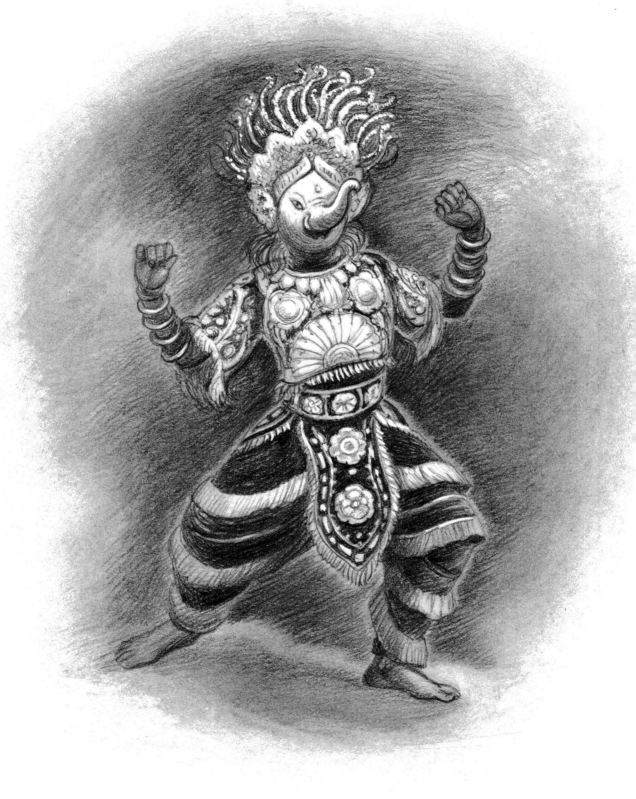

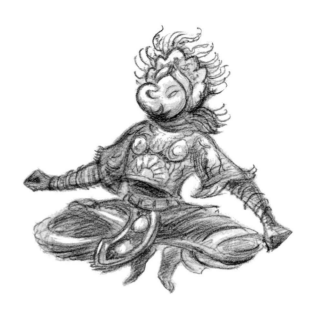

Now at last, stepping down the pathway, glancing sharply from side to side, comes the elephant mask of Ganesha, gleaming white and topped by a shimmering silver crown. Tense, alert, and watchful, he steps into the glare of the lights. For a moment his headdress glitters like a shower of stars, and sparks flash from the silver embroidery and tiny shining mirrors on his black velvet tunic. Then suddenly he is gone, back into the darkness.

He is called by the drummers again and again. He returns, not once but many times. He begins to dance, and with each return he dances with greater strength until he is circling with high leaps that send him spinning around in the air.

Ganesha has no sooner vanished for the last time when the battles begin. Each dance is a drama of battle, signaled by a frenzy of drumming and the shouts of the drummers, joined by the squealing oboe-notes of the *shenai*.

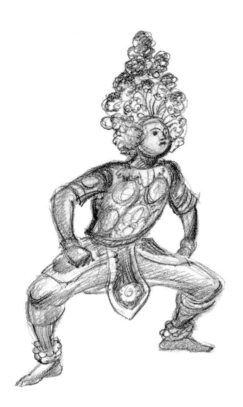

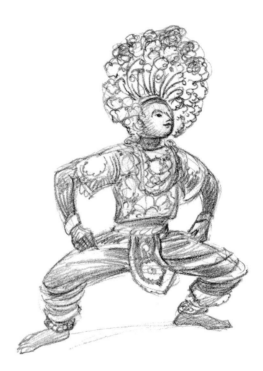

Like Ganesha, the heroes enter with a high-stepping walk and swift glances right and left, their pale masks glimmering under the brightness of their silver crowns. Then they dance faster and faster until they whirl in a circle, spring into the air, and spin around. They land on their knees, and wait, alert and watchful, for their enemy.

He comes, with a fresh burst of drumming, a frightful demon with a snarling face of green or red and a wild mane of hair. Sword in hand, he crouches low on widespread legs. The heroes confront him with violent shaking of their chests and shoulders. Then they spring forward into battle.

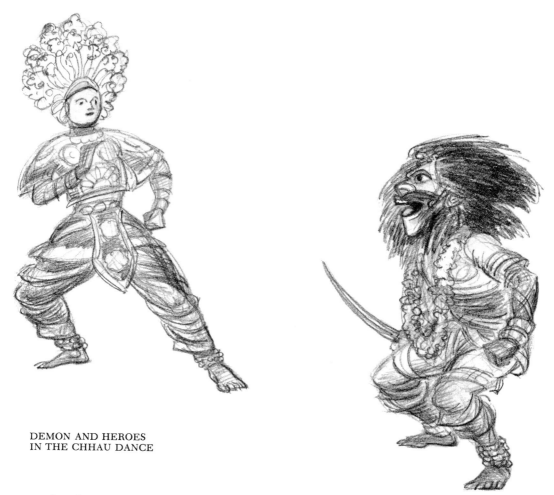

DEMON AND HEROES
IN THE CHHAU DANCE

The drum rhythms change; the drums beat faster and louder as the heroes swirl around their enemy, fighting him not with swords but with waving scarves of white. The demon strikes in vain. At last he falls and lies dying, twitching and writhing on the ground. The heroes circle him in a dance of triumph, then leap away down the path into the darkness and come back again, one by one, somersaulting in the air, rolling over on the earth, and springing high to land upon their knees.

The gods come down to help them fight the demons. Ganesha's brother is the god of war and rides to battle mounted on his peacock steed whose tail spreads out behind him like a fan. The mother goddess Durga slays a buffalo-headed demon that no one else can harm. Krishna, all painted blue, dances with his flute, then turns to do battle with a demon king. Shiva appears as a bearded wise man, and out of the blackness of the night comes the goddess Kali, black-masked and terrible.

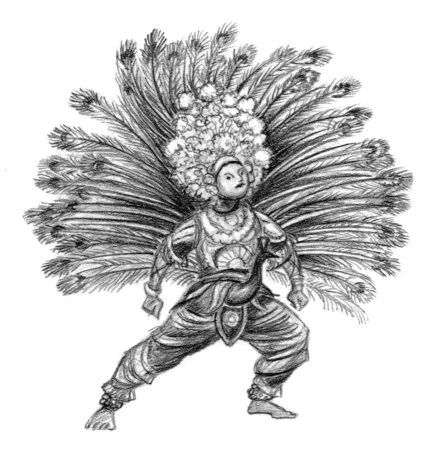

KARTIKEYA, GOD OF WAR, MOUNTED ON HIS PEACOCK

56

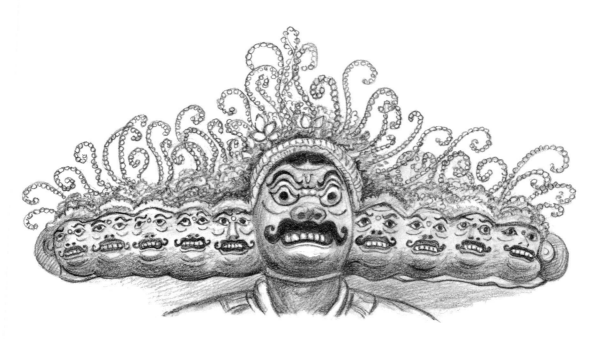

Scenes from the epic of the *Ramayana* come to life in the dusty dancing place. The people press closer to watch the great Rama with his bow, shaking his shoulders in heroic rage; the gallant monkey-general Hanuman; and Ravana, their demon enemy, who carried off Sita to his stronghold far away.

Now a single hero comes prancing in to fight a savage lion, and a huge bear, black and shaggy, joins him in the battle. Dust rises in clouds around them, with an acrid smell like smoke from the mouths of demons. The crowd surges forward in a wave of excitement, spilling over into the dancing place. Men struggle to push the people back, while the bear and lion fight on in the choking dust, the drummers pound their drums like men possessed, and the piercing notes of the *shenai* slice through the shouts of the crowd.

Dancers, musicians, and audience are one. The hundreds of people pressing around the dancing place and the dim figures clinging to the branches of

MASK OF
THE DEMON
RAVANA

the trees above are all part of the drama, the age-old ritual of the spring.

The dark earth and dark sky quiver to the beat of the drums, the stamp of dancing feet. So it must have been when the hunters of long ago danced in the forest and on the hills, the men who painted pictures of masks on the walls of caves and carved them on the naked weathered rocks. They knew, those ancient ones, the mystery of masks, the power of masks to change their wearers into spirits, animals, or even into gods.

The glittering masks of demons, gods, and heroes leaping in the dusty dancing place share with the first masks ever made the same mysterious power. On this festival night, through the power of masks, the gods appear on earth, the demons are slain, and evil is laid low. And after the festival the rains will come.

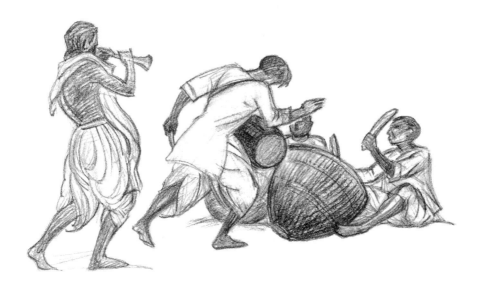

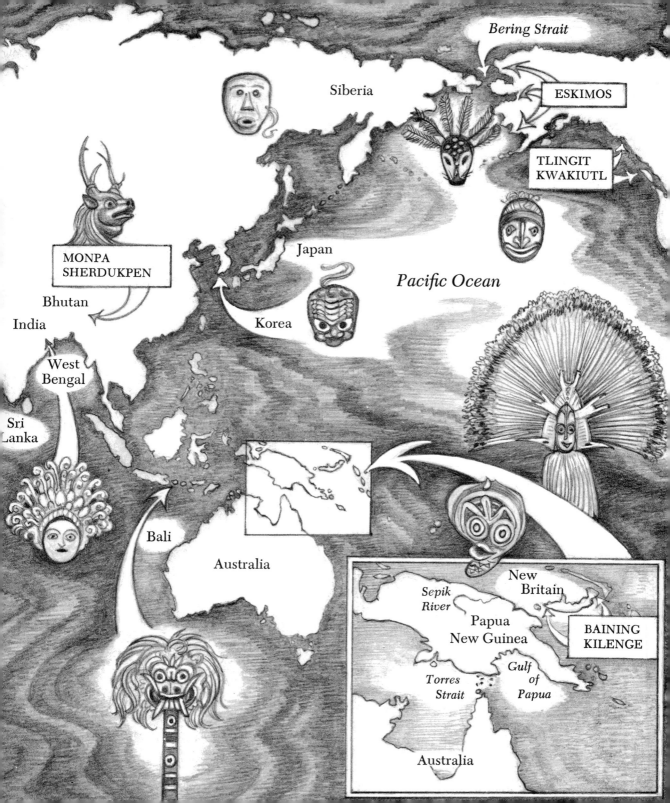

Bering Strait

Siberia

ESKIMOS

TLINGIT
KWAKIUTL

MONPA
SHERDUKPEN

Bhutan

India

West
Bengal

Sri
Lanka

Japan

Pacific Ocean

Korea

Bali

Australia

New
Britain

Sepik
River

Papua
New Guinea

BAINING
KILENGE

Torres
Strait

Gulf
of
Papua

Australia

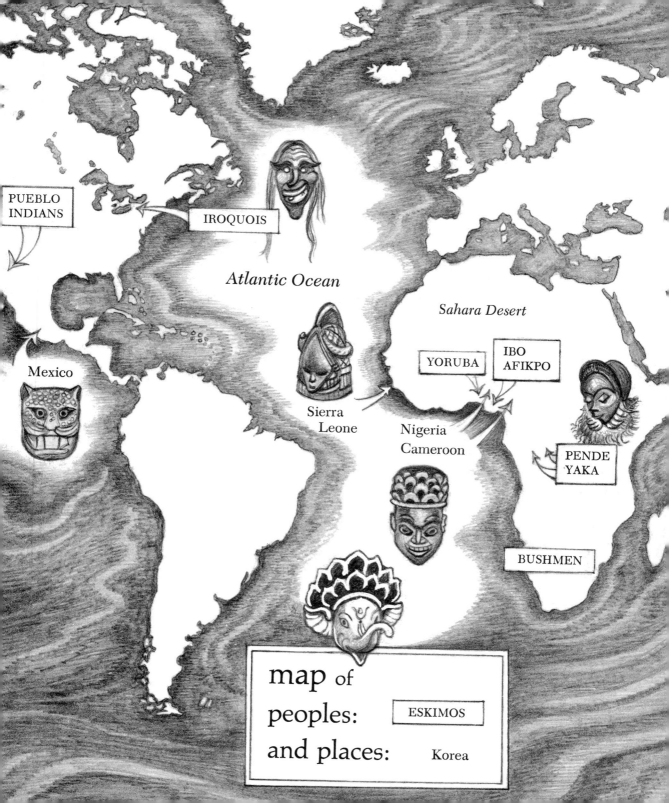

PUEBLO
INDIANS

IROQUOIS

Atlantic Ocean

Sahara Desert

YORUBA

IBO
AFIKPO

Mexico

PENDE
YAKA

Sierra
Leone

Nigeria
Cameroon

BUSHMEN

map of
peoples:
and places:

ESKIMOS

Korea

list of illustrations

The names of some museums have been abbreviated as follows: Robert H. Lowie Museum of Anthropology, University of California, Berkeley—LM; Metropolitan Museum of Art, New York—MMA; Museum of the American Indian, New York—MAI; Sheldon Jackson Museum, Sitka, Alaska—SJM; Smithsonian Institution, Washington, D.C.—SI; UCLA Museum of Cultural History, Los Angeles—UCLA. Page numbers appear in bold type. The measurements of the masks are of height, unless length is indicated.

1 Seal mask. Kuskokwim River, Alaska, Eskimo, 1875–1900. Wood and feathers. 9 in. MAI. **2** (*left*) Mask with two faces and animal head. Lower Yukon River, Alaska, Eskimo, late 19th century. Wood, gut and rawhide. 30½ in. SI. (*right*) Spirit mask. Ogowe River, Gabon, late 19th century. Wood. 9 in. Pitt Rivers Museum, Oxford University. **3** Shaman's mask. Transbaikal region, Siberia, Evenk people, late 19th century. Brass and bearskin. 8½ in. Museum of Anthropology and Ethnography, USSR Academy of Sciences. **4** Mask. Michoacán, Mexico. Gourd. 5¾ in. MAI. **5** (*left*) Mask. Babanki, Cameroon, 1907. Wood. 19 in. Linden-Museum, Stuttgart. (*right*) Mask. Zaire, Luba people. Wood. 14⅝ in. MMA.

the power of masks

6–7 Rock carvings (petroglyphs) from sites in New Mexico. **8** Rock paintings. Hueco Tanks, El Paso, Texas. **9** Kiva paintings. Kuaua Pueblo, Coronado State Park, New Mexico. **10** (*left*) Petroglyphs of masks. Amur River region, Siberia. (*center*) Cave painting of masked figures. Bhimbetka, India. (*right*) Rock painting of masked figure. Tassili, Algeria. **11** (*left*) Bushman painting of masked hunter. Southern Africa. (*center*) Yaqui Indian deer dancer. Mexico. (*right*) Palaeolithic cave painting of dancing shaman in antlered mask. *Les Trois Frères* Cave, Southern France. **12** (*left*) Helmet mask. Zaire, Kuba people. Raffia cloth, cowrie shells and beads. 20½ in. MMA. (*right*) Mask. Blackwater River, Papua New Guinea. Cane basketwork and clay. 22¼ in. MMA. **13** (*left*) Mask for clowning. Papuan Gulf, Papua New Guinea. Bark cloth and cane.

62

UCLA. (*center*) Spirit mask. Kuskokwim River, Alaska, Eskimo, 1875–1900. Wood. 11 in. MAI. (*right*) Shaman's mask. Transbaikal region, Siberia, Evenk people, early 20th century. Iron, cloth and bear fur. 5½ in. Museum of Anthropology and Ethnography, USSR Academy of Sciences. **14** (*left*) Mask for Tlásulá ceremonial dances. British Columbia, Canada, Kwakiutl people. Wood. 11 in. Thomas Burke Memorial Washington State Museum, Seattle. (*center*) Mask for dance and drama, often worn by small boys. Nigeria, Afikpo people. Wood. Collection of Simon Ottenberg. (*right*) Pantomime mask. Arunachal Pradesh, India, Monpa people. Wood. NEFA Museum, Shillong. **15** Ancestor mask. New Guinea (Irian Jaya), Asmat people. Rattan and coconut cord. 80 in. MMA. **16–17** Chhau masks and mask maker. Charida Village, Purulia, West Bengal, India.

e animal world

18 (*left*) Mask for Deer Ceremony. Spiro Mound, Oklahoma, 1200–1600. Wood, shell inlay. 11½ in. MAI. (*right*) Deer dancer. Bhutan. **19** Mask for Deer Dance. Arunachal Pradesh, India, Sherdukpen people. Wood. **20** Yak Dance. Arunachal Pradesh, India, Monpa people. **21** (*left*) Buffalo mask. Ivory Coast, Baule people. Wood. Length: 28 in. University Museum, University of Pennsylvania. (*right*) Buffalo mask. Nigeria, Mama people. Wood. Length: 19½ in. Nigerian Museum, Lagos. **22** (*left*) Horned mask. Zaire, Pende people. Wood. 15 in. American Museum of Natural History, New York. (*center*) Elephant mask with movable jaws. Nigeria, Ogoni people. Wood. Length: 18½ in. British Museum, London. (*right*) Elephant mask. Ivory Coast, Baule people. Wood. 11⅛ in MMA. **23** (*left*) Elephant spirit mask, to be worn on top of the head. Nigeria, Ibo people. Wood. 19 in. Nigerian Museum, Lagos. (*right*) Mask. Erub Island, Torres Strait. Turtleshell, hair and cassowary feathers. 16⅛ in. MMA. **24** (*left*) Fish mask. Orokolo Bay, Papuan Gulf. Bark cloth, cane and grass. 64¼ in. Pitt Rivers Museum, Oxford University. (*right*) Blackfish mask. Lower Yukon River, Alaska, Eskimo, 1890. Wood and feathers. 14½ in. SI. **25** Gannet mask, to be worn sloping over the forehead. St. Michael, Alaska, Eskimo. Wood, gull feathers, eagle down and whalebone. Length: 31½ in. SJM. **26** (*left*) Owl mask. St. Michael, Alaska, Eskimo, 1890–99. Wood and feathers. 6⅝ in. LM. (*right*) Shaman's mask of walrus spirit. Alaska, Eskimo, late 19th century. Wood, ivory and whalebone. 24¼ in. LM. **27** Owl mask. British Columbia, Canada, Kwakiutl people, early 20th century. Wood. 10 in. Thomas Burke Memorial Washington State Museum, Seattle. **28–29** Dancers in the Hamatsa Ceremony. British Columbia, Kwakiutl people. **30** Shaman's mask of bear spirit. Alaska, Tlingit people, 1867. Wood, shell inlay. 10⅝ in. Peabody Museum, Harvard University. **31** (*left*) Ceremonial stone axehead with carving of a man-jaguar. Mexico, Olmec culture, about 800–300 B.C. British Museum, London. (*right*) Jaguar or "tiger" dancer in the drama of the *Tlacololeros*. Guerrero, Mexico. **32** Leopard dancer. Cameroon, Kaka people. **33** Two Egungun masks. Nigeria, Yoruba people. Wood. (*left*) 8⅞ in. (*right*) 26¼ in. UCLA.

64